Delicious Meals for Cheese Lovers

Quick and easy recipes

Author

Kathryn A. Watts

All rights held by Copyright 2021.

DEDICATION

This e-book has been supplied to you for personal use exclusively by the author and publisher. This e-book may not be made accessible to the public in any form. Infringing on a person's copyright is illegal. If you feel the copy of this e-book you're reading violates the author's copyright, please contact the publisher at https://us.macmillan.com/piracy.

Veggie Rice with Smoky Spices 1 Lentil Bowl made with Sweet Potatoes and Cauliflowers Tabbouleh with Sesame, Parsnips, and Wild Rice Bowl of Acai Avocado Dressing for 13 Vegan Kebabs Chilli (15 vegan) 18 Cauliflower Steaks with Olive Salsa and Roasted Red Pepper Salad with Fennel, Roasted Lemon, and Tornato (22 Fennel, Roasted Lemon, and Tornato) Chickpea Salad with No Cooking 28 Black Bean Salad with Guacamole and Mango 31 Vegetables Griddled with Aubergines Melting Bombay Mix of Chickpeas (34 chickpeas) Soup with celeriac, hazelnuts, and truffles (38 Tarka Dhal 40) 47 Vegan Chickpea Curry Jacket Potatoes 50 Veggie Olive Wraps With Mustard Vinaigrette

57 Kidney Bean Curry 61 Avocado Hummus & Crudités 54 Spinach, Sweet Potato & Lentil Dhal With Pecans, 64 Squash & Spinach Fusilli 67 Rice with Artichokes and Aubergines Vegan Tacos in 70 Minutes 7.3 Fritters de Lentil 77 Falafel Recipes That Are Simple To Make Lentil Ragu with Courgetti (80 Lentil Ragu + Courgetti) Lasagne with 84 lentils 87 Peanut Butter Overnight Oats 91 Vegan Shepherd's Pie 96 Chia Pudding with Chocolate 96

Smoky Spiced Veggie Rice

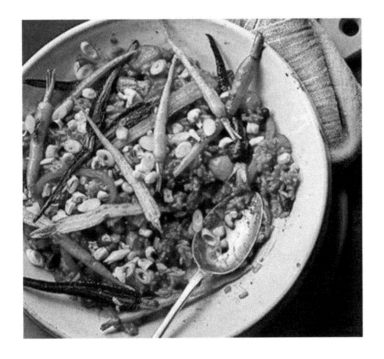

15 rnins to prepare

1 hour. to cook

6 people in a hurry

Try this vegan version of jamb alaya, which is packed with hot and smoky flavors and veggies. It's nutritious, low in fat and calories while yet packing a punch of flavor.

cashews (25 g)

olive oil, 4 tbsp 2 red onions, finely chopped 2 celery sticks, finely chopped 1 com co b 250g rainbow baby carrots, divided lengthways

2 tbsp Cajun seasoning 2 big red peppers, thinly sliced smoked paprika (112 tbsp)

1 teaspoon chipotle aioli tornato purée, 2 tbsp

200g halved heirloom cherry tomatoes drained and washed 400g can kidney beans 400g cherry tomato is es ese ese ese

400ml vegetarian or vegan stock tbsp red wine vinegar 300g long-grain rice, rinsed (vegan varieties are readily available) spring onions, thinly cut 2 tbsp caster sugar

Method

THE FIRST STEP

In a large skillet or casserole dish, dry-fry the cashews until golden brown, about 10 minutes. Remove from the fire and set aside to cool before chopping coarsely. In the same pan, heat 1 tablespoon of oil over high heat and sear the corn for 20 seconds on each side. Remove from the pan and put aside, then add the carrots and continue to cook for another 5 minutes. Set aside after removing it from the pan.

aside.

THE SECOND STEP

In the same pan, put the remaining oil over medium heat and cook the onions and celery for 10 minutes, or until they are soft. delicate and light in color After 5 minutes, add the Cajun spice, smoked paprika, chipotle paste, and tornato purée. Fry for 1 minute at a time till golden brown! After the spices have become aromatic, add the cherry tomatoes and cook for an additional 2 minutes.

THE THIRD STEP

Stir in the kidney beans, canned tomatoes, rice, stock, vinegar, and sugar, and continue to stir until everything is well combined. Everything has been brought together. Bring to a boil, then cover with a!id and reduce to a low heat with a!id. Cook, stirring halfway through, for 35-40 minutes over a medium-low heat, until the rice is cooked and the liquid has been absorbed.

STEP4

Cut the corn from the cob and toss it in with the carrots and rice. Season with salt and pepper and top with cashews and spring onions.

Sweet Potato & Cauliflower Lentil Bowl

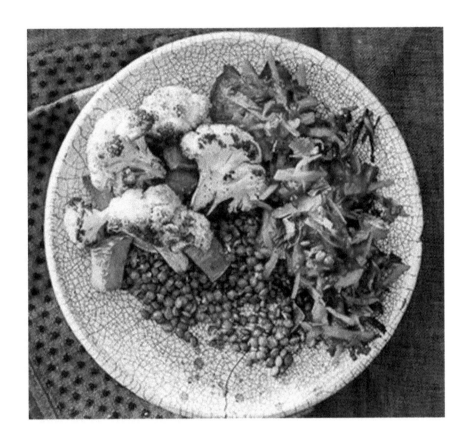

20 minutes to prepare 35-minutes to prepare Serves 4 people.

Make this zesty vegan bowl ahead of time and store it in the fridge for fast, filling lunches whenever you need them. Four of your daily five ingredients are included in each bowlful.

1 big sweet potato, skinned but not peeled, cleaned and sliced into medium chunks 1 cauliflower, sliced into big florets, slivered garam masala (1 tblsp) groundnut oil, 3 tbsp two cloves of garlic
Lentils de Puy, 200g

1 tsp Dijon mustard 1 tbsp th umb-sized slice ginger

2 carrots 14 red cabbage 12 limes, juiced

12 coriander tiny pack

Method

THE FIRST STEP

Preheat the oven to 200 degrees Fahrenheit/180 degrees Fahrenheit fan/gas 6 Toss the sweet potato and cauliflower with the garam masala, a quarter of the oil, and a pinch of salt and pepper. On a large roasting tray, spread out the ingredients. Roast for 30-35 minutes, or until the garlic is soft.

THE SECOND STEP

In the meanwhile, combine the len ti1s and 400ml cold water in a pot. Bring to a boil, then reduce to a low heat and continue to cook for another 20-25 minutes. Although the lentils have been cooked, they still have a bit of a bite to them. Drain.

THE THIRD STEP

Using the biade of your knife, crush the garlic cloves off the tray. Combine the garlic, remaining oil, ginger, mustard, a teaspoon of sugar, and a third of the lime juice in a large mixing bowl. Stir in the heated lentils, season to taste, and X!hisk again. Carrots should be coarsely grated, cabbage should be shredded, and coriander should be roughly chopped. Squeeze the last bit of air out of the

room.

season to taste with lime juice

STEP4

Divvy up the lenti! mi,-xture among four bowls (or four containers if saving and chilling). Serve with a quarter of the carrot slaw and a quarter of the sweet potato and cauliflower combination on each plate.

8

Sesame Parsnip & Wild Rice Tabbouleh

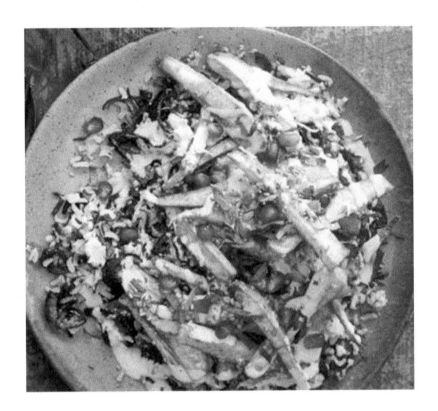

10 minute prep 45-minutes to prepare 3 people

With this quick vegan parsnip & wild rice tabbo uleh, you'll get your fill of flavorful vegetables. Our simple winter salad is flavorful, satisfying, and contains two of your daily five ingredients.

500g (5 medium) peeled and sliced parsnips 2 12 tbsp rapeseed oil (cold pressed) tsp turmeric powder 2 tblsp coriander, ground sesame seeds, 2 tblsp Red onions, diced 130g wild rice

white wine vinegar, 2 tbsp tahini, 3 tblsp
leaves coarsely cut from a small bunch of mint 2 tablespoons pomegranate seeds 1 small bag coriander, coarsely chopped

THE FIRST STEP

Preheat oven to 200°C/180°C fan/gas mark 6. 6. Toss the parsnips with 112 tbsp oil, turmeric, coriander, and a pinch of salt and pepper, then top with sesame seeds. Roast for 30 minutes, or until the vegetables are soft.

THE SECOND STEP

Cook the wild rice according to the package directions in the meanwhile. In a separate pan, heat the remaining 1 tablespoon oil, then add the onion slices and 3 tablespoons water. Cook for 10 to 15 minutes, stirring once in a while, until done! utterly supple Increase the heat to high, add 1 tbsp vinegar, and continue to cook for a few minutes until done! pink flamboyant

THE THIRD STEP

To produce a creamy dr essing, combine the tahini, the remaining vinegar, and just enough warm water. Taste and adjust seasonings as necessary.

STEP4

Drain the wild rice and combine with the onions and 34% of the chopped herbs in a mixing bowl. Distribute among three plates and top with sesame parsnips, pomegranate seeds, and the remaining herbs. Serve with a sprinkle of tahini dressing.

Acai Bowl

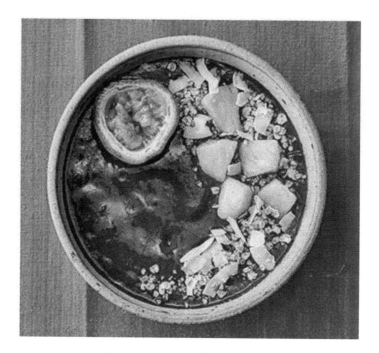

5 minutes to prepare Easy, no-cook

1 portion

For a quick, simple start to your day, try this fruity breakfast smoothie bowl. Toppin gs may be changed according on the season; in the summer, fresh berries or peaches work beautifully.

açai powder (about a teaspoon) frozen grapes from handful
12 ripe banana, cut handful ice cubes, tsp coconut flakes, 5 pineapple chunks, 12 passionfruit, 1 tbsp toasted oats (optio nal)

Method

THE FIRST STEP

In a powerful blender with 100ml water, combine the açai powder, frozen berries, banana, and ice cubes. Blend until smooth, then transfer to a bowl and top with your preferred toppings.

Vegan Kebabs With Avocado Dressing

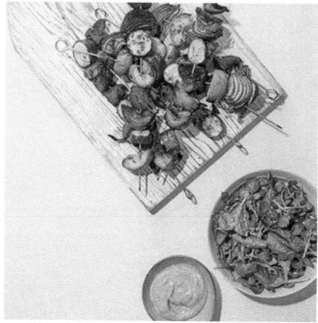

Ingredients

olive o I l 312 tbsp

crushed garLic cloves

1 tblsp chilli powder

freshly chopped ro semary sp rigs

each quartered portobello mushroom 4 quartered peaches, destoned
2 courgettes, sliced into 8 slices each

8 slices each from 2 big red onions (leave the root on) 1 guava

1 freshly squeezed lemon

12 teaspoon mustard, wholegrain

Salad made using a huge bag of rocket, watercress, and spinach toasted mixed seeds (2 tbsp)
You'll need the following:

8 skewers made from metal

Method

THE FIRST STEP

3 tbsp oil, smashed garlic, chili flakes, and rosemary in a mixing bowl Each skewer should include two pieces of mushroom, peach, courgette, and red onion. Set the kebabs aside after brushing them with the flavorful olive oil and seasoning them with salt and pepper. The kebabs may be prepared and stored in the refrigerator for up to a day.

THE SECOND STEP

Preheat the grill or the barbeque to its maximum temperature. Meanwhile, blend the avocado, half the lemon juice, and 50ml water together to make a smooth dressing, seasoning to taste. Toss the combined rocket salaci and toasted seeds with the remaining lemon juice, remaining 12 tablespoons olive oil, and mustard.

THE THIRD STEP

Grill or barbecue the skewers for 4-5 minutes on each side, or until done and slightly browned. Serve with avocado dressing and salaci on the side.

17

Vegan Chilli

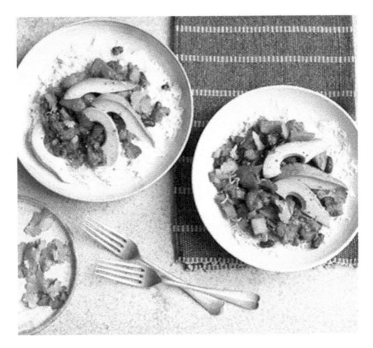

15-minute prep 45-minutes to prepare (or 6 hrs 15 in a slo w coo ke r)

Serves 4 people.
This vegan chili is loaded with veggies and flavor.
For a full meal, combine it with rice or jacket potatoes.

Ingredients

olive oil, 3 tbsp

2 peeled and medium chunked sweet potatoes 2 tsp paprika smoked

1 tsp cumin powder a chopped onion

2 sliced carrots

2 chopped celery sticks 1-2 tsp chilli powder 2 garlic cloves, smashed (depending on how hot you like it) 1 tblsp. oregano (dried)

1 tablespoon pureed tornato

pieces of red pepper

400g chopped tomatoes from a can To serve, combine 400g black beans, 400g kidney beans, drained lime wedges, guacamole, rice, and coriander.

Method

THE FIRST STEP

Preheat the oven to 200 degrees Fahrenheit/180 degrees Fahrenheit fan/gas 3. 6. 1 12 tbsp oil, 1 tsp smoked paprika, and 1 tsp ground cumin drizzled over the sweet potato in a roasting tin Season with salt and pepper and roast for 25 minutes, or until the chunks are cooked.

THE SECOND STEP

In a large saucepan over medium heat, heat the remaining oil. Combine the onions, carrots, and celery in a large mixing bowl. Cook for 8-10 minutes, turning periodically, until the vegetables are tender, then add the garlic and cook for another minute. Toss in the tornato purée and the remaining dry spices. Cook for 1 minute after giving everything a vigorous stir.

THE THIRD STEP

Toss matoes with 200ml water and sliced red pepper. Bring the chili to a boil, then reduce to a low heat and continue to cook for 20 minutes. Before adding the sweet potato, add the beans and simmer for a further 10 minutes. Serve with lime wedges, guacamole, rice, and coriander. Can be frozen for up to three months in an airtight container.
To prepare in a slow cooker, combine all of the ingredients in a large mixing bowl and stir

Over medium heat, heat the oil in a large frying pan. Combine the onion, celery, and shallots in a large mixing bowl. Cook for 8-10 minutes, turning periodically, until the sweet potato pieces are tender, then add the garlic and cook for another minute. Cook for 1 minute, then put into a slow cooker with all the dry spices, oregano, and tornato purée.
Toss in the diced tomatoes and red pepper. Cook on low for 5 hours after stirring everything well. Cook for another 30 minutes to an hour, stirring occasionally. Serve with lime wedges, guacamole, rice, and coriander, as desired.

Cauliflower Steaks With Roasted Red Pepper & Olive Salsa

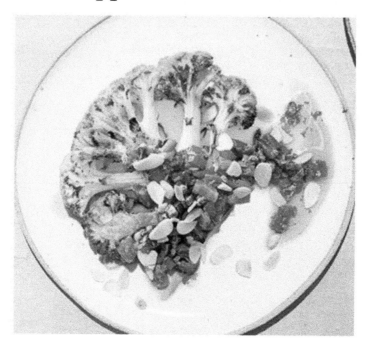

15-minute prep

With a red pepper, olive, and caper salsa and almonds on top, unlock the flavors of cauliflower. It's a delicious light lunch or dinner that's both healthy and vegan.

1 cauliflowe 1 cauliflower 1 cauliflower 1 cauliflower 1 ca

12 tsp paprika smoked roasted red pepper, 2 tbsp olive oil 4 pitted black olives, parsley, tiny handful capers (1 tsp)

red wine vinegar (12 tbsp)

tbsp flaked almonds, roasted

Method

THE FIRST STEP

Preheat the oven to 220°C/ 200°C fan/gas 7 and line a baking sheet with parchment paper. Use the central section of the cauliflower since it is bigger, and preserve the remainder for another time. Season the steaks with paprika and half a tablespoon of oil. Place on a baking sheet and bake for 15-20 minutes, or until well done.

THE SECOND STEP

While you're waiting for the salsa to finish, prepare it. Chop the peppers, olives, parsley, and capers and combine with the remaining oil and vinegar in a mixing bowl. Taste and adjust seasonings as necessary. To serve, ladle the salsa over the steaks and garnish with flaked almonds.

Fennel, Roast Lemon & Tornato Salad

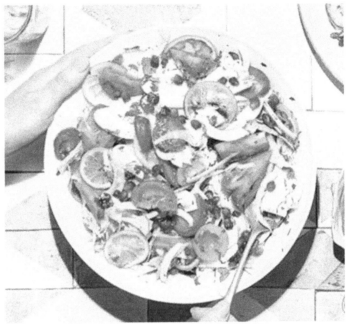

15-minute prep 25-minutes to prepare Easy

6 PEOPLE

To prepare this colorful summer salaci, combine a roasted lemon, fennel fronds, cherry tomatoes, pomegranate, and herbs. It's a great meal to serve to a group of people.

Lemons (two)

500g mixed tomatoes, 1 tbsp extra virgin olive oil, 1 tbsp sugar (I used cherry tomatoes and some larger ones) bulbs fennel

100g seeds of pomegranate

1/.2 tarragon leaves, 1/.2 tarragon leaves, 1 tarragon leaf, 1 tarragon leaf, 1 tarragon leaf, 1 tarragon leaf rnint leaves 1/.2 little pack Method

THE FIRST STEP

Preheat the oven to 200°C/180°C fan/gas 6 and prepare a baking tray with parchment paper. 1 lemon, thinly sliced, put out on baking pan, drizzled with 1/ 2 tbsp oil, and sugar sprinkled on top. Roast for 20-25 minutes, or until shrivelled and caramelized. Keep an eye on them; you may need to remove some of them from the oven before the rest are cloned. These may be prepared the night before and stored at room temperature.

THE SECOND STEP

Roughly cut the tomatoes and finely slice the fennel, reserving the fronds, while the lemons simmer. Combine the remaining olive oil, lemon juice, and pomegranate seeds in a mixing dish. Season with salt and pepper to taste, then toss everything together well.

THE THIRD STEP

When ready to serve, coarsely chop the herbs and combine them with the roasted lemons and fennel fronds in the salad.

27

No-Cook Chickpea Salad

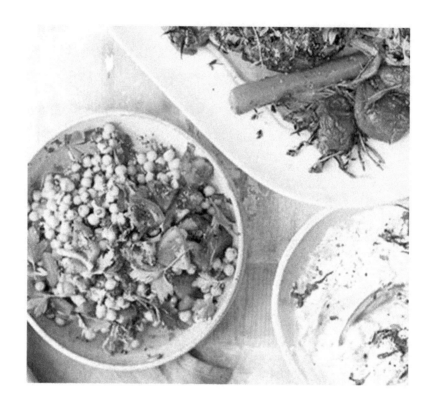

Easy Serves 6 Prep: 10 minutes, no cooking

To liven up a healthful chickpea salad, add a pinch of harissa. It's quick and easy to prepare, and it's the perfect complement to slow-cooked Greek lamb.

400g chickpeas, drained and rinsed small pack coriander, roughly chopped small pack parsley, coarsely chopped red onion, thinly sliced red onion

2 tblsp olive oil 2 big tomatoes, diced

harissa, 2 tbsp

1 freshly squeezed lemon

Method

THE FIRST STEP

Mix all of the ingredients together, pounding the chickpeas a little so that the edges are a little rough - this helps the dressing soak. (Make a day ahead of time and store in the refrigerator.) Serve with tzatziki sauce and slow-cooked Greek lamb.

Guacamole & Mango Salad With Black Beans

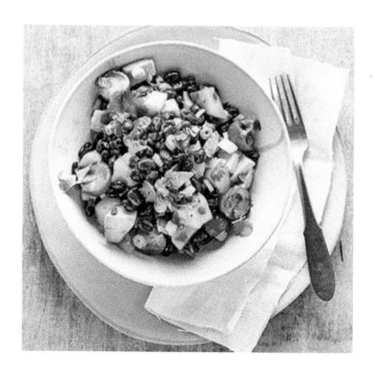

31

15-minutes to prepare Easy to prepare and serve for two people with no cooking required.

With this nutritious salad of mango, avocado, and beans, you'll get four of your five-a-day. It's a nutrient-dense meal that's also gluten-free and vegan.

1 zested and juiced lime

1 mango, peeled, stoned, and cut 100g cherry tomatoes, halved 1 red chilli, deseeded and sliced 1 small avocado, stoned, peeled and chopped

1 finely sliced red onion

12 oz. coriande r, choppe d

drained and washed 400g can black beans

Method

THE FIRST STEP

In a mixing bowl, combine the lime zest and juice, mango, avocado, tomatoes, chilli, and onion. Stir in the coriander and beans.

TIPS FOR COOKING

BEANS IN WATER ARE YOUR BEST OPTION.

Because nothing else is added to canned beans in water rather than brine, you should always select them. Red kidney beans are the next best thing if you can't locate black beans.

33

Griddled Vegetables With Melting Aubergines

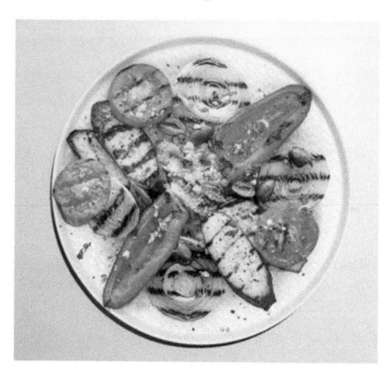

10 minute prep 25-minutes to prepare 2 people Easy

Ali combines five of your five-a-day requirements into a single nutritious vegan meal. It's great griddled on the stovetop or grilled on the grill, and it's flavored with garlic, lemon, and herbs.

Aubergine, big

12 lemon juiced and zested

1 smashed, 2 chopped garlic cloves

1 tbsp parsley, plus more to serve

1 teaspoon extra virgin olive oil, plus a smidgeon for drizzling 4 teaspoons omega seed blend (see tip)
a teaspoon of fresh thyme leaves

1 tbsp (one tablespoon) rapeseedoil

1 quartered red pepper, deseeded

thickly sliced big onion

sliced courgettes at an angle

2 big tomatoes, 3 thick slices each halved 8 Kalamata olives

Method

THE FIRST STEP

Grill the eggplant until it is tender and the skin is bliste red, approximately 8-10 minutes, flipping regularly. Cook it directly over the flame if you have a gas hob. Remove the skin, coarsely cut the flesh, and combine with the lemon juice, 1 minced garlic clove, 1 tablespoon parsley, 1 tablespoon extra virgin olive oil, and the seeds when cool enough to handle. Combine the remaining parsley, garlic, and lemon zest in a mixing bowl.

THE SECOND STEP

In the meanwhile, combine the veggies with the thyme, smashed garlic, and rapeseed oil, preserving the onions as slices rather than rings. Heat a big griddle pan over high heat and char the veggies until they're soft and lines appear - the tomatoes will need the least amount of time. Arrange the aubergine purée and olives on plates, drizzle with extra virgin olive oil, and top with parsley, lemon zest, and garlic.

TIPS FOR COOKING

SEED MIX OMEGA

Seeds supply protein and necessary omega fatty acids in this and other dishes in the Summer 2018 Health and Diet Pian. To prepare the omega seed mix, mix 3 tbsp sesame, sunflower, and pumpkin seeds together in a container, then keep in the refrigerator and use as directed.

37

Chickpea Bombay Mix

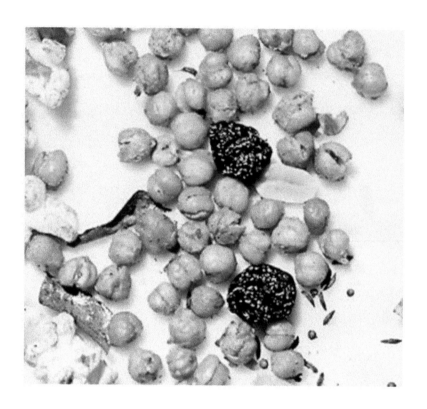

2 minutes to prepare 10 minutes to cook 1 person, simple

When you're craving a snack, whip up this nutritious, gluten-free Bom bay mix. The recipe calls for our curried chickpeas, which you can prepare ahead of time if you have the ingredients on hand.

60 g chickpeas in a curry sauce (see recipe below) 1 tablespoon peanuts (unsalted) raisins (1 teaspoon) Method STEP 1 Combine the unsalted peanuts and the curried chickpeas (recipe here). Bake for 10 minutes at 200°C/180°C fan/gas 6°C, then stir in the raisins.

Tarka Dhal

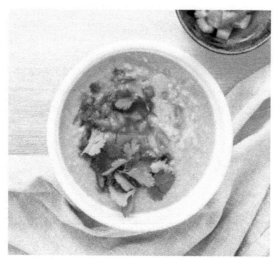

10 minute prep Cooking time: 1 hour 2 servings

When you're cooking on a budget, try this easy dh al for a quick and nutritious s t0r ecupb oard dinner. Use vegetable table oil instead of ghee to make it vegan.

Ingredients

red tiJs 200g

tbsp ghee (or vegan vegetable oil) 1 small onion, coarsely minced garlic cloves

a quarter teaspoon of turmeric (14 tsp)

12 tsp garam masala cori ander
1 chopped smali tornato

Method

THE FIRST STEP

Rinse the le ntils a number of times until they are clean. When the water is clear, put it in a saucepan with 1 litre of water and a pinch of salt. Bring to a boil, then reduce to a low heat and cook for 25 minutes, scraping the froth from the top as needed. Cook for another 40 minutes, stirring regularly, until the mixture has thickened into a soupy consistency.

THE SECOND STEP

While the lentils are cooking, melt the ghee or oil in a nonstick frying pan over medium heat and sauté the onion and garlic for about 8 minutes, or until the onion has softened. Cook for another minute with the turmeric and garam masala added. Remove the item from circulation.

THE THIRD STEP

Pour half of the onion mixture over the lentils in bowls. Serve with tornato and coriander on top.

Celeriac, Hazelnut & Truffle Soup

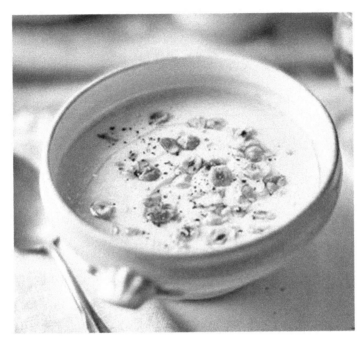

Prep:20 mins
Cook:45 mins
Easy

6 PEOPLE

Serve as a beginning on Christmas Day with this healthful vegan celeriac and hazelnut soup. Leave the truffle oil out for a simple meal on a cold winter night.

In terms of ingredients,

1 teaspoon of extra virgin olive oil thyme sprigs 2 leaves of bay a chopped onion

1 chopped garlic dove

1 celeriac, peeled and diced (about 1 kilogram) 1l veg stock (check the label to make sure it's vegan; we used Marigold) 1 potato (approximately 200g), chopped Soya cream (100 mL) 1 tbsp truffle oil, with an additional drizzle to serve Method S0g blanched hazelnuts, roasted and coarsely chopped

THE FIRST STEP

Heat the oil over a low heat in a big saucepan. Add the onion and a bit of salt to the pan with the thyme sprigs and bay leaves tied together with a piece of twine. Cook for approximately 10 minutes, or until the potatoes are cooked but not brown.

THE SECOND STEP

Cook for 1 mm more after adding the garlic, then add the celeriac and potato. Season with a large teaspoon of salt and white pepper and whisk everything together well. Pour in the stock, bring to a boil, then reduce to a low heat and continue to cook for at least 30 minutes. The veggies are mushy to the point of becoming squishy.

THE THIRD STEP

Remove the herb s, whisk into the cream, turn off the heat, and blitz until completely smooth. Taste for seasoning after each addition of 1/2 tbsp truffle oil; the intensity of the oil varies, so start with less and add a bit at a time.

STEP4

To serve, reheat the soup until it's scorching hot, then spoon it into bowls and top with the hazelnuts, black pepper, and a drizzle of truffle oil on top.

TIPS FOR COOKING

FOR FUTURE USE, FREEZE

Refrigerate for 1-2 days before reheating, or freeze until step 3 is completed. You may make it ahead of time and then thaw and reheat it quickly on a busy day.

Veggie Olive Wraps With Mustard Vinaigrette

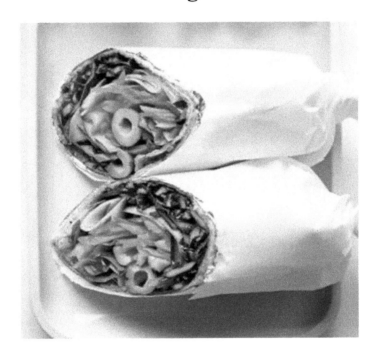

10 minute prep

the absence of a chef 1 person, simple

Our easy, healthful vegetable wrap lets you eat the rainbow. This vegan, low-calorie lunch alternative made with olives and vegetables is perfect for eating on the go.

80 g wedge red cabbage, finely shredded 1 carrot, shredded or coarsely grate thinly cut 2 spring onions
a handful of basi] leaves 1 courgette, shredded or roughly grated
5 pitted and halfed green olives

12 tablespoons powdered English mustard 2 tblsp rapeseed oil (extra virgin) 1 tbsp vinegar (apple cider)
1 big tortilla (with seeds)

Method

THE FIRST STEP

Toss all of the ingredients in a large mixing bowl, except the tortilla. STEP 2 Place the tortilla on a piece of foil and layer the filling down one side of the wrap; it may seem that there is too much filling at first, but it will condense as you roll it tightly. From the filled side, roll the tortilla, folding the edges in as you go. To retain the contents within the wrap, fold the foil at the ends inward. Immediately cut in half and devour. Leave whole and wrap in baking parchment like a cracker if bringing to work.

TIPS FOR COOKING

SWAP INSTRUCTIONS FOR THE INGREDIENTS

Olives aren't your thing? Instead of filling the wrap with the filling, spread it with nut butter like peanut, almond, or cashew. Choose a palm oil-free, sugar-free butter. It will provide more protein, but it will also contribute a bit more fat, so don't overdo it.

49

Vegan Chickpea Curry Jacket Potatoes

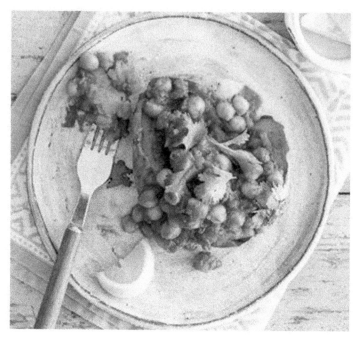

15-minute prep 45-minutes to prepare Easy

4 people

With this delectable chickpea curry jacket, you can add protein to a vegan diet.

It's a flavorful midweek supper or satisfying lunch.
Ingredients

4 potatoes (sweet)

coconut oil (1 tbsp)

12 tablespoons cumin seeds

a chopped big onion

1 smashed garlic clove

1 tsp garam masala 1 tsp thumb-sized piece ginger, coarsely grated

1 tsp coriander, ground

tsp turmeric (12 tblsp.)

tikka masala paste (around 1 tbsp)

2 x 400 g tomato cans, chopped

2 cans chickpeas, 400g each, drained

To serve, garnish with lemon wedges and coriander leaves

Method

P 1 STEP

Preheat oven to 200°C/180°C fan/gas mark 6. 6. Prick the sweet potatoes all over with a fork, then place them on a baking sheet and roast for 45 minutes, or until a knife pierces them soft.

THE SECOND STEP

In a large saucepan set over medium heat, melt the coconut oil. Add the cumin seeds and cook for 1 minute, or until fragrant, before adding the onion and cooking for 7-10 minutes, or until softened.

THE THIRD STEP

Cook for 2-3 minutes in the pan with the garlic, ginger, and green chili. Cook for a further 2 minutes, or until the spices and tikka masala paste are aromatic, before adding the tomatoes. Bring to a simmer, then add the chickpeas and continue to boil for another 20 minutes, or until the sauce has thickened. STE P 4 SEASON n.

Cut open the roasted sweet potatoes lengthwise and serve on four plates. Squeeze the lemon wedges on top of the chickpea curr y. Before serving, season and garnish with coriander.

53

Mexican Beans & Avocado On Toast

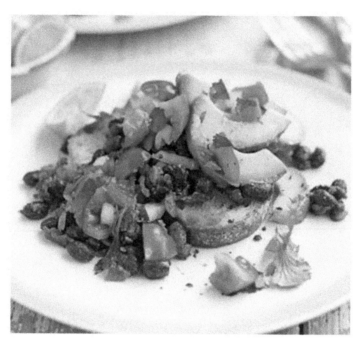

20 minutes to prepare ten minutes to prepare Easy

4 people

Fresh avocado and black beans make a bright Mexican-style breakfast. Make a healthy start for yourself with this simple vegan beans on toast with a twist.

Ingredients

270 grams quartered cherry tomatoes

a coarsely sliced red or white onion

12 lime juice 4 tablespoons olive oil smashed garlic cloves

cumin powder (tsp)

1 teaspoon chipotle paste or chili flakes 4 slices bread 2 x 400g black beans, drained tiny bunch coriander

1 fnely sliced avocado d

Method

THE FIRST STEP

Set aside a mixture of tomatoes, 14 onion, lime juice, and 1 tbsp oil. In 2 tbsp oil, fry the remaining onion until it softens. Fry for 1 minute after adding the garlic, then toss in the cumin and chipotle until fragrant. Pour in the beans and a splash of water, stir to combine, and simmer over low heat until well cooked. Cook for 1 minute after stirring in the majority of the tornato mixture, seasoning well and tossing in the majority of the coriander leaves.

THE SECOND STEP

Drizzle the remaining 1 tbsp of oil over the toast. Place a piece of bread on each dish, followed by a heaping helping of beans. To serve, top with avocado slices and the leftover tornato mixture, as well as coriander leaves.

Spinach, Sweet Potato & Lentil Dhal

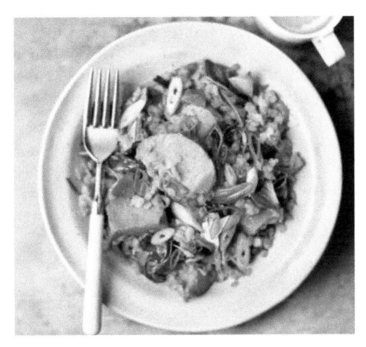

ten minutes to prepare 35-minutes to prepare Easy

4 people

Three of your five-a-day are met with this delicious vegan one-pot dish! This iron-rich, low-fat, low-calorie meal is impossible to go wrong with.

Ingredients

sesame oil (1 tbsp)

a finely sliced red onion 1 smashed garlic clove 1 peeled and coarsely chopped ginger thumb-sized piece a coarsely minced red chili
12 tsp turmeric, ground 1 12 teaspoon cumin powder sweet potatoes, sliced into even slices (approximately 400g/14oz) 600ml vegetable stock, 250g red split lentils spinach pack (80 g)
4 diagonally cut spring onions

12 pac k Thai basi!, ripped leaves

Method

THE FIRST STEP

In a wide-bottomed pan with a tight-fitting cover, heat 1 tablespoon sesame oil. STEP 2 Toss in 1 finely chopped red onion and simmer, turning periodically, over low heat for 20 minutes, or until softened.

THE THIRD STEP

Cook for 1 minute after adding 1 smashed garlic clove, a finely chopped thumb-sized piece of ginger, and 1 finely chopped red chili, then add 1 12 tsp powdered turmeric and 1 12 tsp ground cumin.

STEP4

Increase the heat to medium and add 2 sweet potatoes, sliced into even pieces, stirring to coat the potatoes in the spice mixture.

5

250 g red split lentils, 600 ml vegetable stock, and a pinch of salt and pepper

SECOND STEP

Bring the liquid to a boil, then decrease the heat to low, cover, and simmer for another 20 minutes. The leeks are soft, and the potato is just retaining its form.

STEP7

Season to taste with a pinch of salt and pepper, then fold in the 80g spinach gently. To serve, add 4 diagonally cut spring onions and 12 tiny pack ripped basi! leaves to the wilted spinach.

THE EIGHTH STEP

Allow it cool fully before dividing into sealed containers and storing in the refrigerator for a nutritious lunch.

60

Kidney Bean Curry

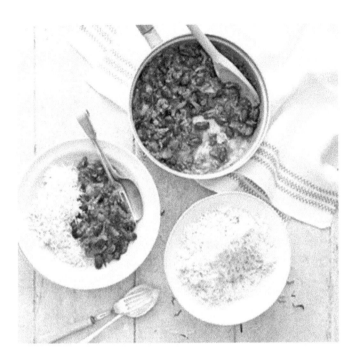

5 minutes to prepare 30 minutes in the oven Easy

2 PEOPLE

When you don't have anything in the fridge and want something quick, tasty, and satisfying, this is the recipe for you.

Ingredients

1 tablespoon oil (vegetable)

diced onion, fine

2 finely chopped garlic cloves

a peeled and coarsely chopped thumb-sized piece of ginger

1 coriander small pack, carefully chopped stalks, shredded leaves 1 tblsp. cumin powder

1 tbsp paprika (ground) garam masala, 2 tsp

Tomatoes, 400g can To serve: 400g canned kidney beans, cooked basmati rice in water

Method

THE FIRST STEP

In a big frying pan, heat the oil on a low heat setting. Cook, stirring occasionally, until the onion is softened and beginning to color, about 10 minutes. Cook for another 2 minutes, until aromatic, with the garlic, ginger, and coriander stems.

THE SECOND STEP

Cook for another minute after adding the spices to the pan, by which time everything should smell fragrant. Bring to a boil with the chopped tomatoes and kidney beans in their water.

THE THIRD STEP

Reduce the heat to low and cook for 15 minutes, stirring occasionally. The curry has a wonderful, thick consistency to it. Serve over basmati rice and coriander leaves after seasoning to taste.

63

Avocado Hummus & Crudités

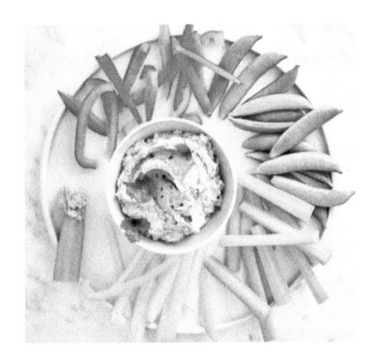

10 minute prep

o Prepare

Simple

2 PEOPLE

This healthy, low-calorie vegan food may be served as a lunch or a starter. Enjoy this delectable avocado-based hummus.
Ingredients

1 peeled and seeded avocado 210 grams drained chickpeas
1 d ove d ove d'ove d'ove d'ove

a pinch of chilli flakes (plus a little more to serve)

freshly squeezed lime

coriander leaves by the handful 2 carrots, sliced into strips Method: 160 g sweet snap peas

THE FIRST STEP

Blitz the avocado, chickpeas, garlic, chili flakes, and lime juice together in a food processor until smooth. Season with salt and pepper to taste. Serve the hummus with carrot, pepper, and sugar snap crudités, as well as coriander leaves and a few extra chilli flakes on top. Make ahead of time for a delicious lunch to take to work.

66

Squash & Spinach Fusilli With Pecans

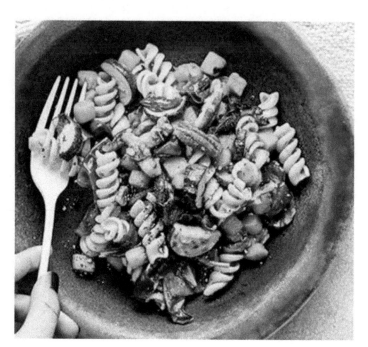

10 rnin s rnin rnin rnin rnin rnin Easy to prepare in 40 minutes

2 PEOPLE

This colorful low-fat, low-calorie squash and spinach pasta with pecans is suitable for non-vegans. In gredients, it's both delicious and healthy.

1 tablespoon chopped sage leaves 160 g butternut squash, diced 3 garlic cloves, sliced large courgette, halved and sliced 2 tablespoons rapeseed oil 6 halves pecan
11 gram fusilli wholemeal STEP 1: Preheat oven to 350°F. 125g bag baby spinach

Preheat oven to 200°C/180°C fan/gas mark 6. 6. Toss the butternut squash, garlic, and sage in the oil, then spread in a roasting tin and bake for 20 minutes. Add the courgettes and bake for another 20 minutes.

15 minutes more to cook Stir everything together, then add the pecans and continue to cook for another 5 minutes until everything is done. The vegetables are tender and beginning to caramelize, and the nuts have been toasted.

THE SECOND STEP

Meanwhile, cook the pasta according to the package directions, which should take around 12 minutes. Drain, then toss with the spinach in a serving bowl to wilt it in the pasta's heat. Add the roasted vegetables and pecans, tossing well before serving, breaking up the nuts a little.

69

Artichoke & Aubergine Rice

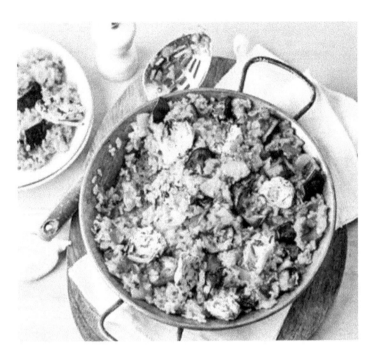

15-minute prep 50 minutes in the oven Easy

6 PEOPLE

This aubergine and artichoke dish is low fat, low calorie, and cost efficient, in addition to being delicious. Make a big quantity and enjoy it cold the following day.

olive oil, 60 mL

pieces of aubergine 1 big finely chopped onion 2 smashed garlic cloves small pack parsley leaves, stems neatly chopped 2 tsp paprika smoked
turmeric, 2 tblsp

Paella rice is 400 grams.

Kallo vegetable stock (12 liters)

chargrilled artichokes (packs of 17Sg)

Lemons (two) 1 sliced into wedges for serving, 1 juiced

Method

THE FIRST STEP

In a large nonstick frying pan or paella pan, heat 2 tablespoons of the oil. Fry the aubergines until they are attractively colored on both sides (adding another tbsp of oil if they start to catch too much), then remove and put aside. In the same pan, add another tbsp of oil and softly cook the onion for 2-3 minutes, or until it has softened. Cook for a few minutes more with the garlic and parsley stems, then add the seasonings and rice and mix thoroughly. Heat for 2 minutes, then add half of the stock and simmer for 20 minutes, uncovered, over medium heat, stirring periodically to avoid sticking.

THE SECOND STEP

Place the aubergine and artichokes in the mixture, pour in the remaining stock, and continue to simmer for another 20 minutes, or until the rice is done. Chop the parsley leaves and season with salt and pepper. Bring the whole skillet to the table and ladle into bowls, garnishing with lemon wedges.

Easy Vegan Tacos

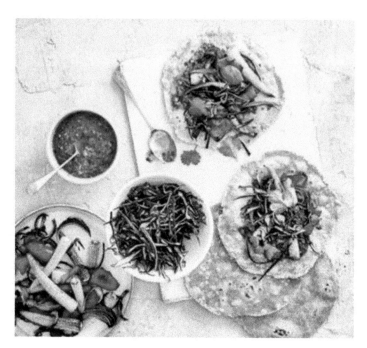

Coo k:30

minutes Prep:1

rnin s Prep:1

rnin s

Preparation:1

rnin s

Preparation:1

Easy

2 PEOPLE

Make vegan tacos with a smoky-sweet salsa for a filling weekend meal. The salsa
takes on a moreish, fruity character thanks to the kiwi.

Ingredients

Baby corn in a 175g bag

1 big, sliced red onion (190g)

1 deseeded, coarsely chopped red pepper

a quarter teaspoon of cumin seeds rapeseed oil (two teaspoons)
1 ripe kiwi, cut in half lengthwise (110g) 1 tornato, cut in half (11Sg)
100g wholemeal flour, plus a little more for rolling

a huge clove of garlic

1 teaspoon chopped fresh coriander

vegan bouillon powder (tsp)

12 tsp paprika smoked

85 g finely shredded red cabbage

Method

THE FIRST STEP

Preheat the oven to 220°C/200°C fan/gas 7 Toss the corn, red onion, and pepper with the cumin seeds and olive oil in a wide shallow roasting pan. Roast for 20 minutes with the kiwi and tornato on one side of the pan.

THE SECOND STEP

In the meanwhile, prepare a dough by mixing 60ml water into the flour with a knife. Knead quickly until smooth, then divide into four equal pieces and roll each out into a 16cm circular tortilla on a lightly floured board. To prevent drying, cover with a tea towel.

THE THIRD STEP

Return the vegetables to the oven for 10 minutes after removing the cooked tornato and kiwi from the pan. Remove the peel from the kiwi and combine the meat, tornato, garlic, half of the coriander, bouillon, and paprika in a mixing bowl. Blitz to a smooth salsa using a hand blender.

STEP4

Cook the tortillas one at a time in a big nonstick fryin g pan without oil for a minute on one side and approximately 10 seconds on the other side, until done. They inflate out a bit, as you can see.

Spread some salsa on a tortilla, then pile on the cabbage and roasted vegetables, finishing with the rest of the coriander. Eat with your hands after adding a dollop of salsa.

76

Lenti! Fritters

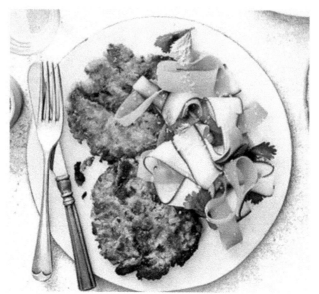

15-minute prep ten minutes to prepare 2 people Easy

With our basic lentils recipe, courgette, and carrots, you can make the delicious lentil fritters in about 25 minutes. They're nutrient-dense, low-fat, and low-carb.

Ingredients

leftover 300g a handful of chopped coriander, lenti ls, lenti ls, lenti ls, lenti 1 onion, finely chopped

2 carrots, courgettes, 50g gram flo ur

12 tsp sesame seeds coriander leaves

1 lime, 12 tablespoons sesame oil

rapeseed oil (1 tblsp)

Method

THE FIRST STEP

Set aside the remaining lentils, together with the chopped coriander, spring onion, and gram flour. Cut the carrots and courgettes into long ribbons with a peeler, then mix them in sesame oil and lime juice with the sesame seeds and coriander.

THE SECOND STEP

Using a frying pan, heat the rapeseed oil. Place four lenti dollops on top! To make the patties, combine all of the ingredients in a large mixing bowl and shape into patties. Serve with the ribbon salad after frying each side until browned.

79

Easy Falafels

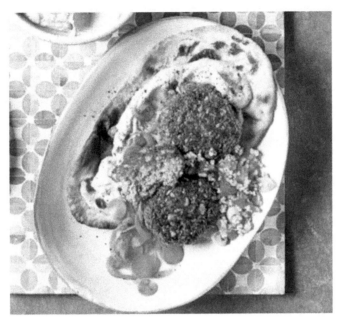

15-minute prep 20 minutes of cooking time + at least 8 hours of soaking time E asy

16th

For a fantastic meze of a meal or a sharing beginning, combine John Torode's simple falafels with soft flatbreads, well-seasoned humous, and crisp pickles.

Ingredients

250 g dry split broad beans or dried chickpeas

12 teaspoon soda bicarbonate 3 cloves garlic
1 chopped onion 1 celery stalk, coarsely chopped 1 leek

1 tiny chilli, finely chopped (deseeded if you don't like it spicy) tsp cayenne pepper 1 tsp cumin 1 tsp sumac 1 tbsp coriander (chopped) parsley, chopped in a large handful

100ml vegetable oil (80g gram flour) Houmous, tabbouleh, and pickled red onion and radish (see goes well with), flatbreads, store- bought or see goes well with (optional)

Method

THE FIRST STEP

Soak chickpeas for 8 hours or overnight in cold water. STEP 2 In a food processor, pulse the chickpeas with the bicarb until smooth. d. d. d. d. d. d d Set aside about a third of the mixture.

THE THIRD STEP

Purée the remaining mixture in the processor to a paste with the garlic, veggies, spices, and herbs. Add the gram flour, season, and stir well to incorporate the paste into the rough purée of chickpeas.

STEP4

Preheat oven to 110 degrees Fahrenheit/ 90 degrees Fahrenheit fan/ 1 degree Fahrenheit gas. Pour some of the oil into a large nonstick frying pan and heat over medium heat. Form the mixture into patties using your hands (there sho uld be enough to make about 16). Cook for 2 minutes on each side or until golden brown. While you sauté the rest of the mixture, keep it warm in the oven by adding a little oil to the pan with each batch. Serve with houmous, tabbouleh, and pickled red onion and radish, if desired, wrapped in flatbreads.

TIPS FOR COOKING THIS RECIPE REQUIRES SOAKED DRIED BEANS; canned beans will not work in this recipe.

Lentil Ragu With Courgetti

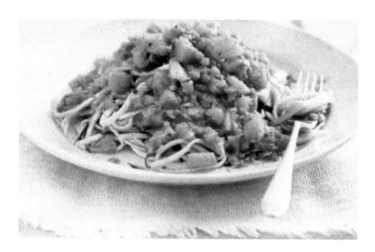

15-minute prep 40-minutes to prepare Easy

4–6 people

A tornato 'pasta' dish that makes the most of your spiralizer. This five-a-day vegan meal will fill you up to the brim.
Ingredients

3 celery sticks, diced 2 carrots, chopped 1 tbsp rapeseed oil, plus 1 tbsp

2 onions, coarsely chopped 140g button mushrooms from a 280g box, quartered 500g dry red lentils 500g passata

11 vegetab le bouillon ed-salt reduc (we used Marigold) 1 tblsp. oregano (dried)
balsamic vinegar, 2 tablespoons

1 or 2 big courgettes, spiralized, julienned, or sliced into noodles with a knife

Method

THE FIRST STEP

In a large sauté pan, heat 2 tbsp of oil. Fry for 4-5 minutes over high heat, until the celery, carrots, garlic, and onions soften and begin to color. Fry for another 2 minutes with the mushrooms.
THE SECOND STEP

Combine the lentils, passata, bacon, oregano, and balsamic vinegar in a large mixing bowl. Cover the pan and cook for 30 minutes on low heat! Tender and pulpy lentils Check and stir periodically to ensure the mL'Cture doesn't cling to the bottom of the pan; if it does, a drop of water should be added.
THE THIRD STEP

In a second frying pan, heat the remaining oil, then add the courgette and stir-fry gently to soften and warm through. Half of the ragu should be served with the courgetti, and the remainder should be saved to enjoy later. It is possible to freeze it for up to three months.

TIPS FOR COOKING

FREEZE

This recipe serves a large number of people, although any lef tover ragu freezes nicely.

Lentil Lasagne

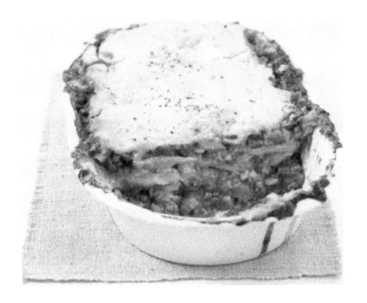

15-minute prep

1 hour 15 minutes to prepare Easy

4 people

This vegan bake utilizes cauliflower and soy milk for the white sauce and canned lentils for the filling.

1 teaspoon of extra virgin olive oil

1 chopped onion

1 sliced carrot

1 celery stick, peeled and finely chopped

d ove d'ove d'ove d'ove d'ove

lentils, drained and rinsed from two 400g cans 400g cornflou r 1 tbsp cornflou r 1 tbsp cornflou r 1 tbsp cornflou r 1 tbsp cornflou r 400g corn

1 tsp ketchup with mushrooms

1 teaspoon oregano, finely chopped (or 1 tsp dried)

1 teaspoon powdered vegetable stoc k

Cauliflower heads, shattered into florets

9 dry egg-free lasagnesheets 2 tablespoons unsweetened soya milk pinch freshly grated nutmeg

THE FIRST STEP

In a pan, heat the oil, then add the onion, carrot, and celery, and gently cook for 10-15 minutes, or until the vegetables are tender. Cook for a few minutes after adding the garlic, then add the lentils and cornflour and mix to combine.

THE SECOND STEP

Toss in the tomatoes, along with a can of water, the mushroom ketchup, oregano, stock powder, and salt and pepper to taste. Cook, stirring periodically, for 15 minutes at a low heat.

THE THIRD STEP

In the meanwhile, cook the cauliflower for 10 minutes or until soft in a pan of boiling water. Using a hand blender or food processor, purée the beans with the soya milk. Add the nutmeg and season thoroughly.

THE FOURTH STEP

Preheat the oven to 180 degrees Celsius/160 degrees Celsius fan/gas 4. A third of the le nti should be spread out! Pour the mixture into the bottom of a 20 x 30 cm ceramic baking dish. Cover with a single layer of lasagna, snapping the edges together.

fit the sheets Spread a third of the lentil mixture on top, then a third of the cauliflower purée, then a layer of spaghetti. Finish with the remaining purée and the final third of lentils and lasagna.

5

Cover loosely with foil and bake for 35-45 minutes, removing the cover for the last 10 minutes.

90

Vegan Shepherd's Pie

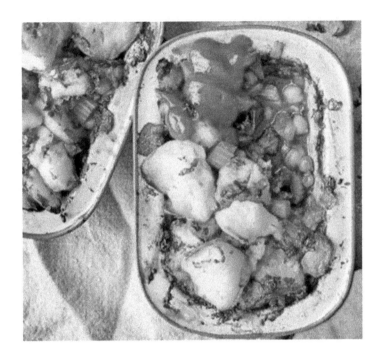

30 Minutes to prepare

1 hour 20 minutes to prepare

If preparing two big pies, cook time will be 1 hour and 45 minutes.

Easy

8 people (makes eight individual] or two large pies)

Porcini mushrooms, leeks, carrots, and butternut squash are combined in this cozy vegan meal, which is finished with crispy potatoes. It's low in calories and fat, and it's ideal for the cooler months.

1 pound floury potatoes (Maris Piper or King Edward) veggie oil, 50 mL
30g porcini mushrooms, steeped for 15 minutes in boiling water and then drained (reserve the liquid)
2 sliced large leeks

2 tblsp. chopped onions

4 medium carrots, chopped into tiny cub es (about 300g)

(make sure it's vegan; we used Kallo) vegetarian stock cube tbsp tornato purée 3 garlic cloves (crushed) 2 tsp paprika smoked

peeled and cut into tiny cubes 1 small butternut squash

12 little bag marjoram or oregano, chopped leaves

12 leaves from a tiny bag of thyme

12 tiny bunches sage, finely cut leaves 4 chopped celery sticks
300g frozen peas 400g canned chickpeas olive oil (20 mL)
tornato ketchup, little box flat-leaf parsley (optional) Method
THE FIRST STEP

In a large saucepan, combine the unpeeled potatoes, water, and salt. Bring to a boil, then reduce to a low heat and cook for 40 minutes, or until the potatoes are tender. Skins begin to separate. Allow to cool somewhat after raining.

THE SECOND STEP

93

In a big heavy-based sauté pan or flameproof casserole dish, heat the vegetable oil in the meanwhile. Cook, stirring occasionally, for 5 minutes, until the mushrooms, leeks, onions, carrots, and stock cube have softened. Reduce the heat and stir more often, scraping the pieces from the bottom of the pan if it begins to stick. Soft but not mushy vegetables are preferred.

THE THIRD STEP

To the rnato purée, add the garlic, paprika, squash, and herbs. Cook for 3 minutes, stirring occasionally, before adding the celery and cooking for a few more minutes.

THE FOURTH STEP

In a large mixing bowl, combine the chickpeas, water from the can, and mushroom stock that has been set aside. Stir in the spinach and peas until well combined. Season, turn off, and put aside after 5 minutes of cooking, stirring periodically. There should always be enough liquid, and the vegetables should be vibrant and crisp.

P 5 (STE)

Remove and discard the skins from the potatoes. 200g of potato should be mashed with a fork and mixed in with the vegetables. Season the remaining potatoes with the olive oil and parsley after breaking them into chunks s, m, and i.

P 6 STEP

Fill the pie pans halfway with filling, then top with potatotes. Preheat the oven to 190°C/170°C fan/gas 5°C and bake the pies for 40-45 minutes, or until golden brown. The filling is warm and the top is golden.

gh Check after 20 minutes if creating individuai pies. As with every good shepherd's pie, it's best served with tornato ketchup.

Peanut Butter Overnight Oats

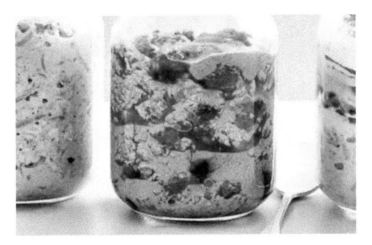

5 minutes to prepare

Plus, there's no need to cook it since it's been soaking overnight.

1 portion

With creamy peanut butter and tart raspberries, make an indulgent but healthy dish of overnight oats. Make it ahead of time and bring it to work in a jar.

Ingredients

80 g raspberry puree, frozen 0g porridge oats (rolled) a tablespoon of maple syrup peanut butter (tbsp)

Method

THE FIRST STEP

Combine the frozen raspberries, 150 mL water, and a teaspoon of salt in a mixing bowl, then cover and chill overnight.

THE SECOND STEP

Combine the maple syrup and peanut butter the following day, then top the oats with it.

Chocolate Chia Pudding

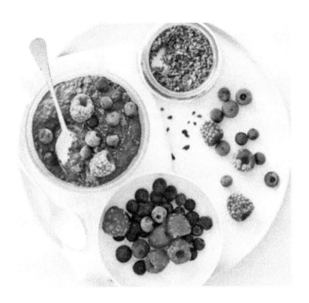

5 minutes to prepare

There's no need to prepare, and
it just takes four hours to cool

4 people

In five minutes, you can make a delicious, nutritious chocolate pudding. It's also low in calories and vegan, and chia seeds are high in omega-3 fatty acids.
Ingredients

chia seeds (60 g)

400 mL almond or hazelnut milk (unsweetened). tbsp maple syrup + 3 tbsp cacao powder

12 tsp vanilla extract cacao nibs, mixed frozen berries, to serve

In a large mixing basin, whisk together all of the ingredients with a good sprinkle of sea salt. Refrigerate for at least 4 hours, preferably overnight, after covering with cling film.

EP 2 (ST)

Place the frozen berries and cacao nibs on top of the pudding in four glasses.

CPSIA information can be obtained
at www.ICGtesting.com
Printed in the USA
LVHW060746221221
706918LV00008B/382